TRAVEL YOGA

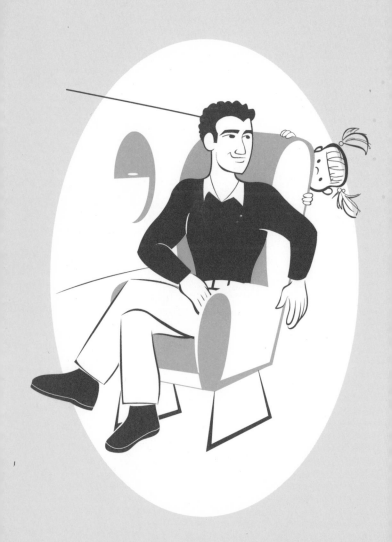

TRAVEL YOGA

STRETCHES FOR PLANES, TRAINS, AUTOMOBILES, AND MORE!

by **Darrin Zeer**

illustrations by **Frank Montagna**

CHRONICLE BOOKS
SAN FRANCISCO

Text copyright © 2005 by Darrin Zeer.
Illustrations copyright © 2005 by Frank Montagna.
All rights reserved. No part of this book may be reproduced in
any form without written permission from the publisher.

Library of Congress Cataloging-in-Publication Data available.

ISBN 0-8118-4503-6

Manufactured in China
Designed by Brooke Johnson

Distributed in Canada by Raincoast Books
9050 Shaughnessy Street
Vancouver, British Columbia V6P 6E5

10 9 8 7 6 5 4 3 2 1

Chronicle Books LLC
85 Second Street
San Francisco, California 94105
www.chroniclebooks.com

CHOOSE THE ROAD
LESS TRAVELED....

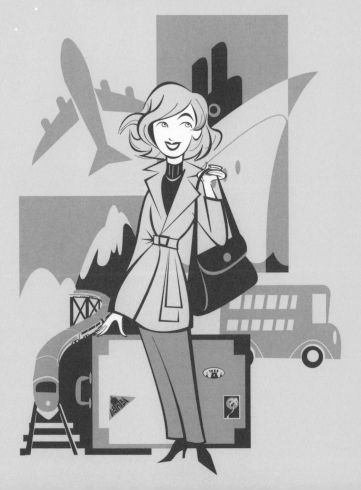

CONTENTS

QUICK HELP GUIDE

INTRODUCTION

✈ *Travel Yoga* is your perfect
guide to a stress-free journey.

Whether your trip is for business or pleasure, practicing yoga is your ultimate relaxation tool. Don't worry—you won't need to stretch your body like a pretzel, and you don't need any prior yoga experience to receive benefits. In fact, the tighter and tenser you are, the more this book is meant for you. You can practice these easy and relaxing exercises whether you're sitting in a cramped airplane seat, waiting in a long line, resting in your hotel room, or jet-setting around the globe—wherever and whenever you might need a little calm.

Before we start, it's important to understand a bit about yoga. Yoga is a practical path to inner peace and wisdom that originated in India over five thousand years ago. It consists of hundreds of stretching exercises that create health and well-being. And because travel requires so much waiting and waiting and waiting, you'll have plenty of time to practice these stretches, no matter how overwhelmed you feel.

So let's get started! This guide is organized into five parts: "Packing Peace of Mind," "Arrival and

Departure Patience," "Stretching in Planes, Trains, Boats, and Automobiles," "Relaxation in Your Home Away from Home," and "Yoga Around the Globe." All together, this little handbook offers over sixty quick and easy techniques to combat stress throughout your trip. So go ahead: flip through the pages and dive in. If you have a specific ache or pain, turn to the "Quick Help Guide" on page 7. And if you can't take the book with you on your travels, be sure to pull out the card at the back and toss it into your bag for instant relief.

You've now booked your ticket to the ultimate peaceful travel adventure.

Happy travels!

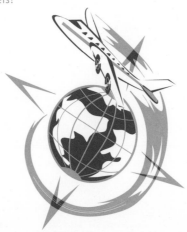

5 KEYS TO HAPPY TRAVELS

1. Be patient—master the art of waiting.

2. Be friendly to your fellow travelers; kindness has many rewards.

3. Find pleasure in your travel experience; it will make any bumps along the way more tolerable.

4. Practice stretching and relaxation exercises throughout your journey; they will transform your trip.

5. Take things one step at a time. When stressed, simply take a deep, relaxing breath for instant peace of mind.

PHILOSOPHY OF THE ENLIGHTENED TRAVELER

Imagine standing in the middle of a busy airport terminal and feeling completely at ease. It's possible! With the help of yoga, you can teach yourself to stay calm, no matter how stressful your surroundings are.

The enlightened traveler's first reaction to all stressful situations is "No problem. I am calm." When a challenge that seems to have no solution arises, the enlightened traveler thinks, "No problem. I am calm." Because the enlightened traveler stays calm in all situations, she or he finds it easier to solve problems and let wonderful experiences unfold.

Remember that travel is more fulfilling when you manage your stress level. You can spend your travel time in either worry or wisdom. Think about this the next time you're in line or delayed. If you feel anxious, a state of calm is just a stretch and a deep breath away. Make a commitment here and now that peace of mind will be your highest priority throughout your trip.

The rewards of the journey far outweigh the risk of leaving the harbor.

—Anonymous

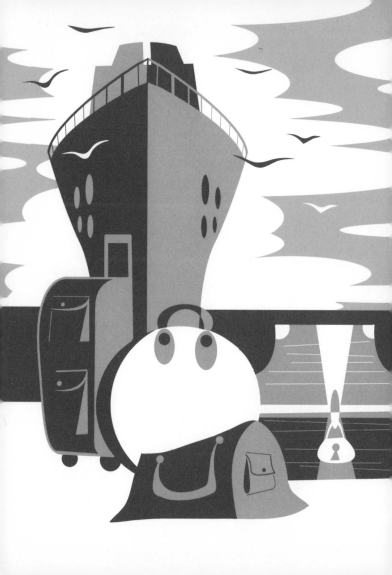

READY,
STRETCH,
GO!

1

Packing Peace of Mind

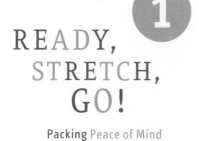

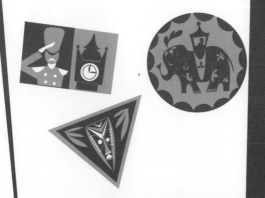

PAIN-FREE PACKING

Getting ready for your trip need not be stressful! The secret is to start a few days before your departure. Whenever you think of an item you'll need, toss it into your suitcase, or at least add it to your packing list. It's also fun to invite a friend to help you brainstorm what you need to bring and even to help you fold and pack your stuff. For a complete packing reminder list and for special Travel Yoga items, please refer to page 94 at the back of the book. Use a backpack as your carry-on, so that both of your arms can be free to practice Travel Yoga without any strain.

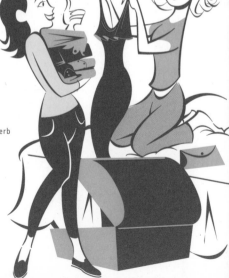

On a long journey even a straw weighs heavy.
—Spanish proverb

HOME CLEAN HOME

No one likes to come home to a mess. So whether you're leaving for the day or for a month, give your abode a once-over. Make the bed, water the plants, clear the clutter, and—most important—wash the dishes! Think of this as a special gift to yourself, an inviting way to return home.

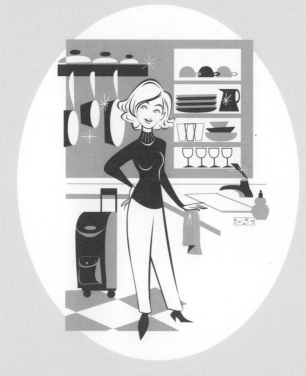

Lugging baggage can be a pain—literally. And long flights, car rides, and train trips can stiffen up your body. So indulge in this soothing stretch series to prepare yourself for the journey ahead.

CAT AND COW POSE

- ✳ Your hands should be directly beneath your shoulders and your knees directly beneath your hips.

- ✳ Inhale as you slowly raise your head and arch your lower back downward. Point your tailbone to the ceiling.

- ✳ Exhale as you slowly drop your head and arch your lower back upward.

- ✳ Repeat five to ten times or as many as time allows.

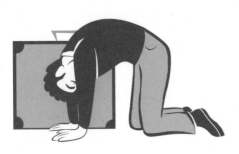

A person who walks in another's tracks leaves no footprints.

–Anonymous

HEAVY SUITCASE STRETCH

* As you lie on your back, slowly bend your legs at a ninety-degree angle.

* Plant your feet firmly on the ground beneath your knees.

* Put your arms at your sides with your palms down.

* Gently raise your hips off the ground to a comfortable height.

* Breathe, hold for fifteen seconds, release, and repeat.

Patience is the best remedy for every trouble.
—Titus Maccius Plautus

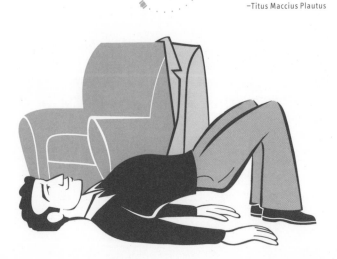

GENTLE COBRA

* Lie flat on your stomach, with your forearms flat on the ground.

* Keep your elbows touching the sides of your ribcage.

* Keep your hips on the ground and your buttocks tight to support your lower back.

* Gently lift your head and chest with the strength of your back.

* Breathe and stretch; feel the strength of your back muscles.

* Hold this stretch for fifteen seconds, then release and repeat.

CHILD'S POSE

* Sit back on your calves, lean forward, and rest your upper body on your legs.

* Let arms rest at your sides. Turn your face to one side.

* Let your body relax, and breathe deeply.

* Repeat this mantra: "I will stay calm and patient throughout my journey."

INNER ITINERARY

Before you jump into the fray at the terminal, work out a game plan. Make sure your possessions are organized and handy, with your ID and travel documents easily accessible. When you arrive, pause before you step out of the vehicle, take a deep breath; the journey has just begun. And remember: The most important part of your plan should be to arrive early. This will allow plenty of time to practice Travel Yoga.

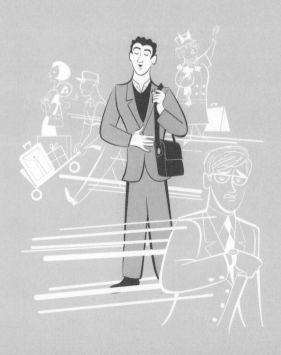

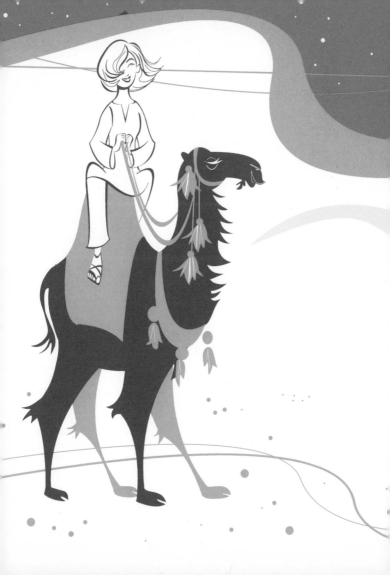

NATURAL WONDERS *of the* WORLD
MEDITATION

Relax . . . breathe . . .

      imagine getting lost in the Sahara Desert.

  Travel through the vast emptiness;

      all is quiet, a gentle wind blows,

your worries simply fall away,

      you let the stillness take over.

Have a vision not clouded by fear.
      —Cherokee proverb

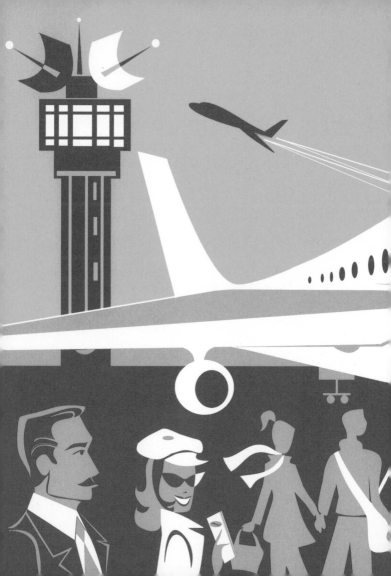

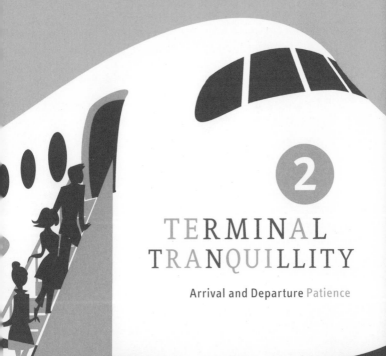

2

TERMINAL
TRANQUILLITY

Arrival and Departure Patience

For most of us, standing in line is nerve-wracking, especially when we're in a rush. The following exercises will help you limber up and take your focus off your wait.

PATIENCE POSE

- ☀ Standing on your left foot only, cross right foot over left. Right toes should not touch the ground.

- ☀ Put your hands on your waist and focus your gaze on a spot a few feet in front of you.

- ☀ Feel the sole of your left foot rooted into the floor, balance on your left leg, and feel your posture rise upward.

- ☀ Take five deep breaths while focusing on being patient, and then switch legs.

Start by doing what is necessary, then do what is possible, and suddenly you are doing the impossible.
—St. Francis of Assisi

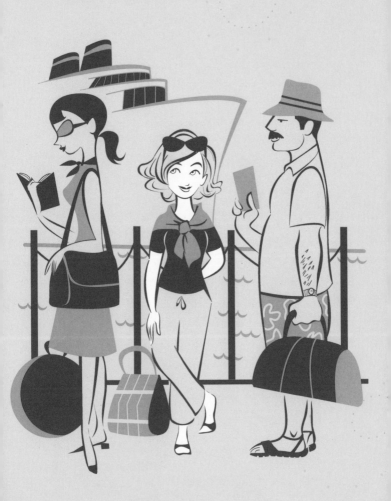

STEADY STANDING POSTURE

- ❋ To ease strain on your lower back, stand with your feet hip-width apart and knees slightly bent.

- ❋ Imagine a string pulling upward at the crown of your head. Feel your spine lift into a straight line.

- ❋ Let your shoulders relax downward and back, soften your jaw, relax your forehead, lower your chin, and don't forget to breathe.

- ❋ To help yourself stay calm, breathe in and out in a slow, steady rhythm.

- ❋ Notice that when your chest rises outward, your back immediately straightens, you naturally take a deep breath, and your shoulders and neck rise and align.

Can you feel the difference? This simple shift in posture improves not only your physical well-being, but also your mood.

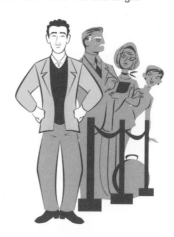

LOOSEN-UP POSE

* Place your hands on your hips.

* With your legs hip-width apart, bend both knees slightly.

* Make wide, full circles with your hips, and remember to smile.

* Next, place your hands on your lower back, fingers pointing downward.

* Tighten your buttocks and stretch your upper body backward.

* Breathe and relax into the stretch.

Life is not so short but that there is always time for courtesy.
—Ralph Waldo Emerson

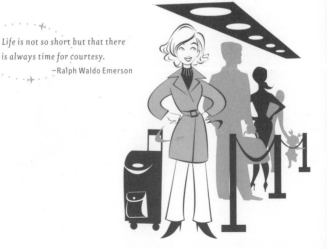

CHEERFUL CHEST OPENER

* Interlace your fingers behind your back, bend forward and slowly raise your arms.

* Let your chest rise, and breathe into the stretch.

* Take five deep breaths and then gently release your arms.

* With loose fists, gently pound on your lower back.

* Don't forget to share a smile with those around you.

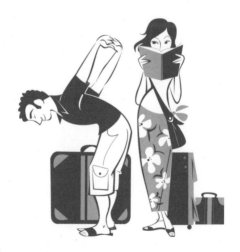

The best way to cheer yourself up is to cheer everybody else up.

–Mark Twain

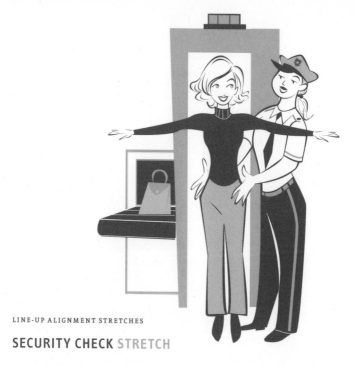

LINE-UP ALIGNMENT STRETCHES

SECURITY CHECK STRETCH

* Hold your arms straight out to the sides.

* Stretch your fingertips toward the opposite walls.

* Pull your hands in opposite directions and let your shoulders relax.

* Breathe, relax, and smile!

RANDOM ACTS OF PATIENCE

Security personnel have one of the toughest jobs in travel. They have to be hypervigilant and eagle-eyed while exercising extreme patience. Patience goes a long way, as does a simple smile and a "Thank you very much." Your random acts of patience will help you stay calm and bring a smile to those who serve you.

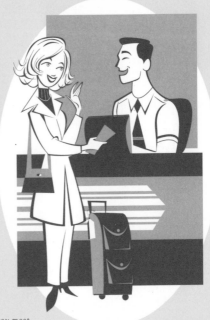

Be kind, for everyone you meet
is fighting a hard battle.

–Plato

Waiting is a large part of the travel experience. So why not use this time to practice Travel Yoga? Stretch your body, soothe your mind, and savor the moment.

FLIGHT-GOT-BUMPED RAG DOLL STRETCH

- ❀ While sitting, reach your hands toward the sky.
- ❀ Breathe in deeply, and relax completely on the exhalation.
- ❀ Drop your arms and upper body toward the ground like a rag doll.
- ❀ Breathe deeply.
- ❀ Stay here until you feel refreshed.

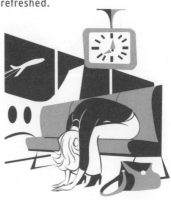

Courage consists of the power of self-recovery.

–Ralph Waldo Emerson

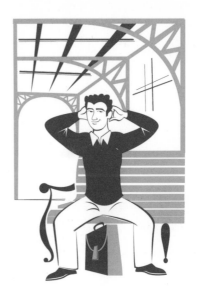

HAPPY TRAVELS STRETCH

* While sitting, interlace your fingers behind your head.

* Relax your elbows and shoulders.

* Smile, breathe, and stretch your elbows backward.

* Feel your shoulder tightness releasing and your chest opening.

* Repeat this calming exercise as needed.

LAYOVER LOWER BACK RELIEF

- ✳ Lie on your back and slide your legs up against the wall.

- ✳ Rest your hands on your belly and close your eyes.

- ✳ Feel your lower back loosen.

- ✳ Breathe and forget about your hurries and worries.

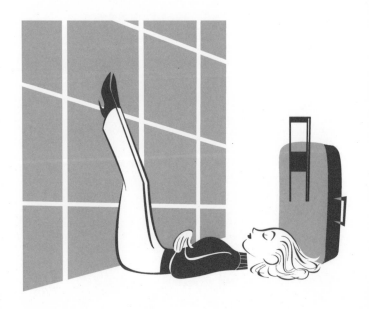

ADVANCED BACK SUPPORT

❀ Stand with your back and palms flat against the wall.

❀ Slowly walk your feet out in front of you.

❀ Use your hands to slow your descent as your back slides down the wall.

❀ Lower yourself until you are in a sitting position with your thighs parallel to the floor, knees at a ninety-degree angle, and feet directly below your knees.

❀ Do not let your knees extend beyond your toes.

❀ You will feel your buttocks and legs getting a great workout.

❀ Hang in there, and don't forget to breathe.

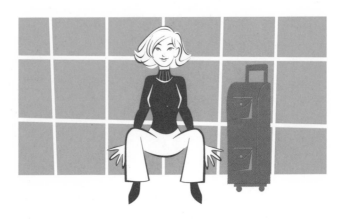

Pressurized cabins, turbulence, recycled air, and long hours of sitting can leave you feeling groggy upon arrival. These Arrival Revival stretches will get your circulation going and soothe sore muscles.

GET A GRIP!

* ❋ Tightly interlace your hands and rotate hands in wide circles.

* ❋ Massage and squeeze hands together.

* ❋ Release hands and shake them.

* ❋ Curl fingers into a tight claw, into a tight fist, and then stretch fingers wide apart.

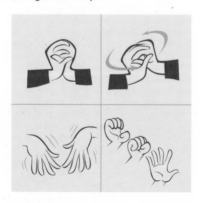

What would life be if we had no courage to attempt anything?
    —Vincent van Gogh

SERVICE STATION REJUVENATION

* Shake your hands and arms vigorously.

* Shake each leg and foot, one at a time.

* Swing your arms in wide circles– up and around and from side to side. Switch directions.

* Wiggle your whole body till it feels loose.

* Raise your arms above your head.

* Reach your hands toward the sky and rise onto your toes.

* Breathe, stretch, and feel your whole body reenergize!

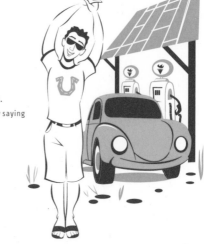

Man plans . . . God laughs.
—Old Hebrew saying

GROUNDING TREE POSE

* Stand next to a table or chair for balance.

* Place your right foot against the inside of your left thigh.

* If your foot slides down, place your right hand on it.

* If you feel steady, put your hands against your chest in prayer position.

* Feel the standing foot rooted into the ground.

* Relax and breathe.

* Stand straight and balanced. Switch legs slowly.

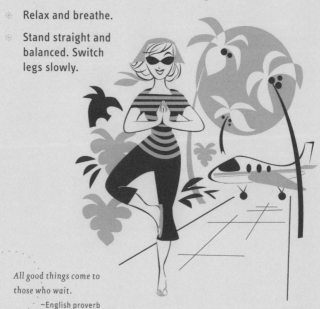

All good things come to those who wait.
—English proverb

LAST LEG OF THE TRIP LEG BENDS

- ❊ Place your hand on a solid surface to steady yourself.
- ❊ Keeping your back straight, squat down slowly for a moment.
- ❊ Take a deep breath, then slowly rise.
- ❊ Repeat this move several times, breathing in rhythm.
- ❊ Try this with your feet flat or balancing on the balls and toes of your feet.

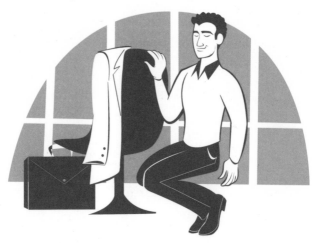

The world is a book, and those who do not travel read only a page.

—St. Augustine

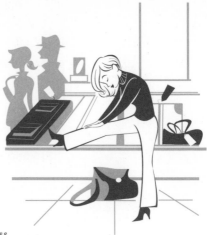

LUGGAGE CAROUSEL LUNGE

* Lift your right foot onto a solid bench or table.

* Turn your standing foot to the side for balance.

* Stretch over your right leg, placing your hands on your leg or on the table.

* Drop your head and breathe into the stretch.

* Flex your foot. Breathe.

* Relax your foot. Breathe.

* Switch legs and repeat.

He who would travel happily must travel light.
—Antoine de Saint-Exupéry

NATURAL WONDERS *of the* WORLD
MEDITATION

Breathe . . . relax . . .

imagine journeying into the Grand Canyon.

Soar into its depths, inhale the fresh air,

lose yourself in the majestic beauty.

Find calm in the canyon!

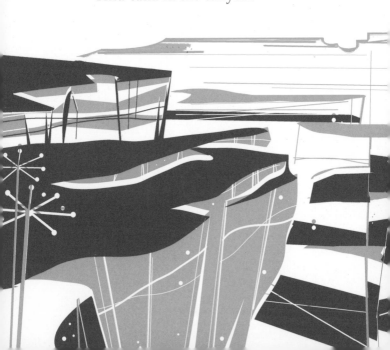

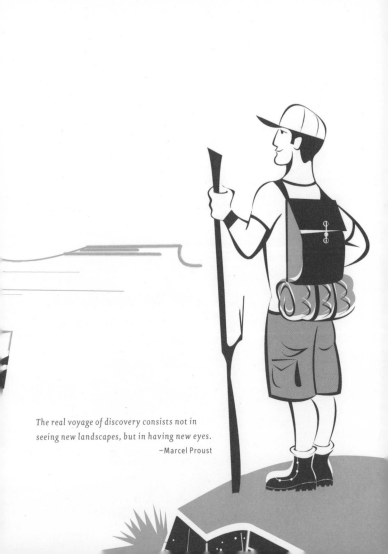

The real voyage of discovery consists not in seeing new landscapes, but in having new eyes.

—Marcel Proust

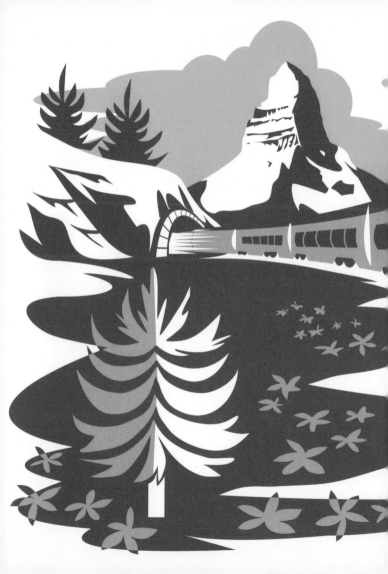

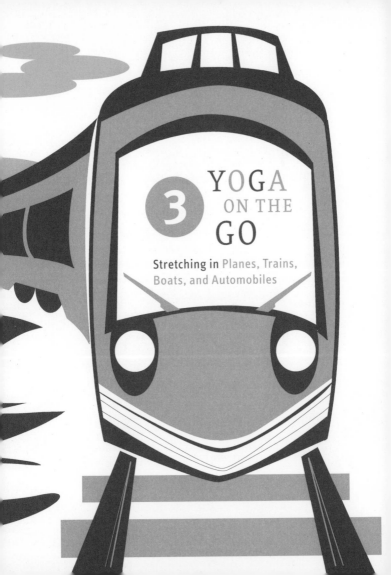

3 YOGA ON THE GO

Stretching in Planes, Trains, Boats, and Automobiles

Try the stretches in this section as you are getting settled into your seat. They will help you get comfy and prepare you for the next step of your journey.

SITTING SURVIVAL

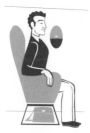

❋ First, sit on your sit bones; to find these sharp bones, place your hands under your buttocks and rock forward and backward until your weight is on these two bones.

❋ Notice that when you rise forward, your body aligns atop your sit bones; your back straightens, your chest expands, and your shoulders, neck, and head rise and align.

❋ Now sit back on your tailbone—everything slumps and drops, including your mood!

❋ Rise forward again. Feel your spine lift into a straight line all the way up to your head, and hold.

❋ Let your shoulders relax, soften your jaw, lower your chin, and take a few deep, calm breaths.

Courage is like love, it must have hope for nourishment.

—Napoléon Bonaparte

GETTING A LEG UP STRETCH

- ❋ While sitting, interlace fingers below one knee.
- ❋ Bend leg up toward your chest.
- ❋ Stretch forehead to knee. Hold and breathe.
- ❋ Switch legs.

CROSSED LEG TWIST

- ❋ While sitting, cross your left leg over your right.
- ❋ Place your right hand or elbow on the crossed knee.
- ❋ Gently turn your body to the left and look behind you.
- ❋ Switch legs and twist the other way.

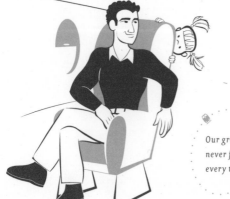

Our greatest glory is not in never falling, but in rising every time we fall.
—Confucius

FRIENDLY NEIGHBOR POSE

- ✳ Sit near the edge of your seat with your arms on the armrests, holding the sides with your hands.

- ✳ Gently stretch your chest up and forward and tilt your head slightly backward.

- ✳ Relax and breathe into the stretch.

- ✳ Then slouch down and let your head drop forward.

- ✳ Feel your spine rolling forward and backward with each stretch.

- ✳ When you're done, smile and introduce yourself to your neighbors.

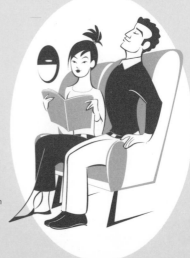

We are all travelers in the wilderness of this world, and the best we can find in our travels is an honest friend.
–Robert Louis Stevenson

This stretch series works on all modes of transportation—planes, trains, buses, and ferries. It's amazing what a bit of stretching can do to bring relief!

PAIN IN THE NECK RELIEF

HEAD ROLLS

- ❋ Slowly roll your head around in a wide circle in both directions.

- ❋ Find a tight spot and stop.

- ❋ Hold and breathe, letting your breath release the tightness.

SHOULDER ROLLS

- ❋ Raise your shoulders to your ears, hold, breathe, and then drop.

- ❋ Roll one shoulder and then the other in wide circles in both directions.

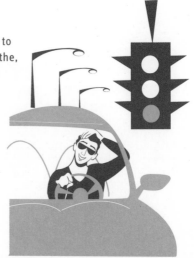

ARM BEHIND BACK

* Stretch your left arm behind your back.

* Grab your wrist with your right hand.

* Drop your head to the right.

* Roll head slightly and explore any tightness.

* Stretch and breathe.

* Repeat with other arm.

ARM ABOVE HEAD

* Bend your left arm above and behind
  your head.

* Grab your elbow with your
  right hand and
  stretch upward.

* Breathe and let
  shoulders relax.

* Repeat with
  other arm.

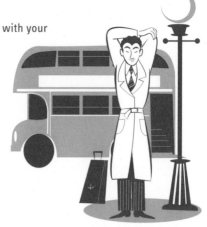

MILE-HIGH MASSAGE

NECK AND SHOULDERS

* Place both hands on your shoulders and neck.

* Squeeze with your fingers and hold for a moment or two.

* Rub vigorously in circles while keeping shoulders relaxed.

WRISTS AND FOREARMS

* Wrap one hand around the opposite forearm.

* Squeeze the muscles with thumb and fingers.

* Move up and down, from your elbow to fingertips and back again.

* Repeat with other arm.

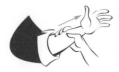

Worry often gives a small thing a big shadow.
—Swedish proverb

TURBULENCE TENSION TAMER

When turbulence hits, let your shoulders drop, relax tight muscles, and release facial tension. Remind yourself to breathe slowly, and focus your attention on your breath. Make the out-breath two times longer than the in-breath. This will immediately calm you.

❋ Repeat this mantra: "I am calm."

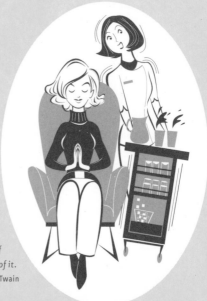

*Courage is not the lack of
fear. It is acting in spite of it.*
—Mark Twain

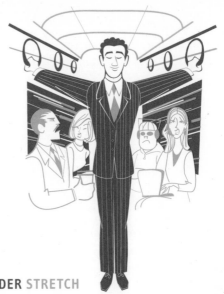

STANDING SHOULDER STRETCH

- ❋ Grab onto something solid about shoulder height to either side. If you're on the bus, the poles work well. If you're on a plane or train, try the overhead compartments.

- ❋ Gently let your body lean forward and your chest stretch outward.

- ❋ Relax your head and breathe.

- ❋ Feel the nice stretch in your chest and shoulders.

Two great talkers will not travel far together.
—Spanish proverb

At the end of the journey, you may feel stiff and tense. These pre-landing stretches are sure to loosen you up and get your circulation flowing.

LEG LOOSENER

❋ Tighten your tummy, straighten your legs as much as you can, and lift them half an inch off the ground.

❋ Let your chest rise, and push your elbows into your seat-back.

❋ Stretch your toes forward.

❋ Rotate your feet in both directions.

❋ Repeat whenever you feel lethargic. You will disembark refreshed and ready to get back on the move.

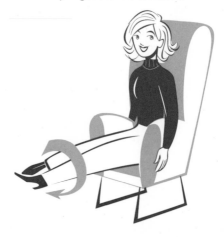

ARRIVAL WARM-UP

* Sit forward with your feet flat on the ground.

* With hands on hips, relax your shoulders and let them drop.

* Rotate your torso in wide, slow circles.

* Breathe and relax as you explore the tightness.

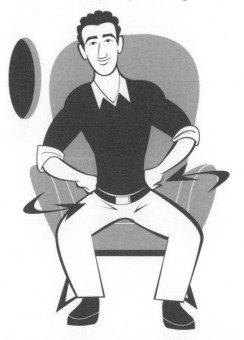

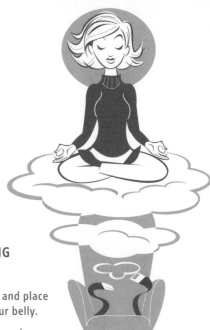

PEACEFUL LANDING
MEDITATION

* Close your eyes and place one hand on your belly.

* Let your shoulders drop.

* Breathe slowly and deeply.

* Feel your hand rise and fall.

* Allow a gentle feeling of relaxation to flow through your body.

* Repeat this mantra: "I am calm and patient."

Patience is the companion to wisdom.

—St. Augustine

OVERHEAD LUGGAGE REACH

Try not to rush off the plane with everyone else; it will just stress you out and ultimately save you only a moment or two. Before reaching for your bags in the overhead compartment, take a moment to stretch and regroup.

* Raise your arms straight above your head.

* Interlace your fingers.

* Alternately turn palms downward and upward.

* Stretch from the ribcage and breathe deeply.

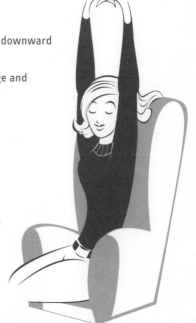

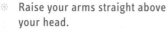

When you reach the end of your rope, tie a knot in it and hang on.

—Thomas Jefferson

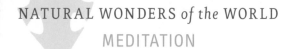

NATURAL WONDERS *of the* WORLD
MEDITATION

Breathe . . . relax . . .

imagine getting lost in the Amazon jungle.

Breathe in the fragrant air,

listen to the vibrant life singing,

let the river carry you into a

deep and peaceful state of mind.

For my part, I travel not to go any-
where, but to go. I travel for travel's
sake. The great affair is to move.
—Robert Louis Stevenson

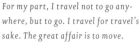

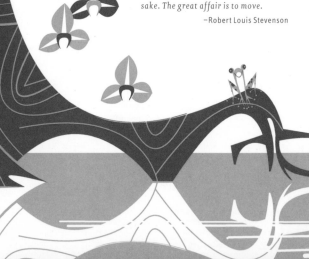

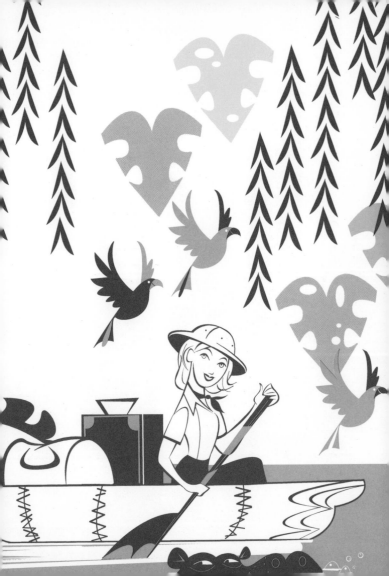

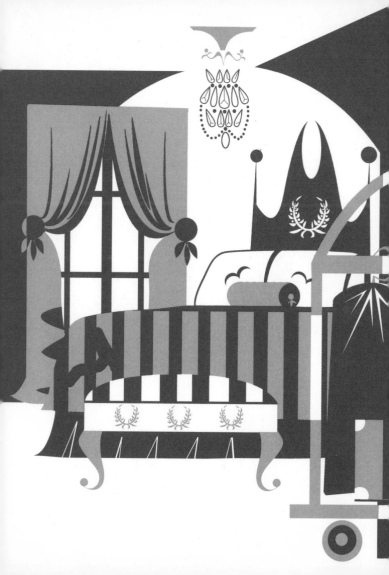

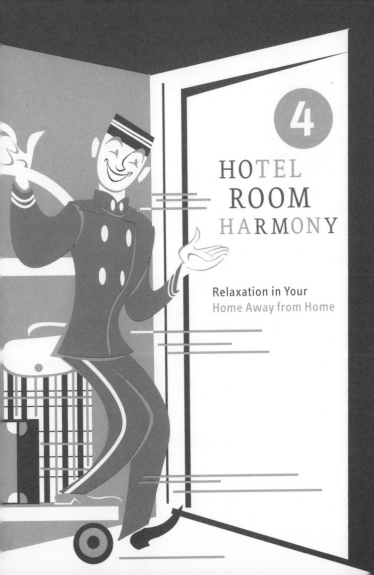

4

HOTEL ROOM HARMONY

Relaxation in Your
Home Away from Home

Make your hotel room a home away from home. The following exercises will bring comfort to any space.

TRAVEL ALTAR

Claim your room as your own by setting up a personalized altar. Pick the best spot on your table or bureau and clear all advertisements off it. Set family photos, candles, and special mementos for inspiration. When you feel frazzled or far away from your loved ones, spend time looking at your altar to rekindle fond memories of home.

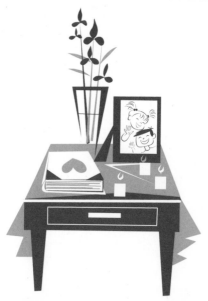

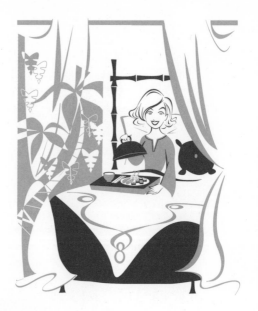

ROOM SERVICE ROYALTY

Splurge once in a while. You're worth it! Order room service. Choose a good movie or some nice music and chill out. Get cozy with your pillows propped up to comfortably support your head and back. Slowly, deliberately eat your meal, and enjoy every bite.

Love can turn the cottage into a golden palace.

—German proverb

SPA NIGHT

- ✳ Unpack your travel spa kit. (Refer to "Travel Yoga Packing Reminders" on page 94 for ideas on things to bring.)

- ✳ Light some candles and incense.

- ✳ Put on some music.

- ✳ Make sure the temperature in your room is cozy warm.

- ✳ Fill the bathtub with warm water and add bath salts and aromatherapy oils.

- ✳ Sink deeply into the tub and let any tension drift away. Take some time to count the many blessings in your life.

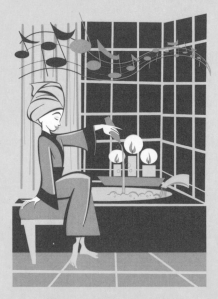

These stretches will help you feel calm and energized before your day gets started.

SUNRISE SOOTHER

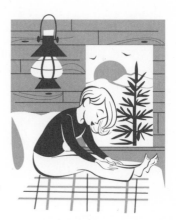

* Lie comfortably on your bed and bring both knees to your chest and wrap your arms around them.

* Drop both knees to one side, arms out to the sides, keeping your shoulders flat; relax into the stretch.

* Gently bring both legs back up, and switch sides.

* Knees at your chest again, rock back and forth.

* If you can, sit up into a forward bend, legs out and upper body stretching forward.

* Take hold of your legs. Relax your shoulders and drop your head.

* Take several deep full-body breaths, stretching a little farther each time. Don't push it.

We are what we repeatedly do. Excellence, then, is not an act, but a habit.
—Aristotle

VACATION SALUTATIONS

This gentle series of yoga postures will help wake up your entire body. Take the first round slow and easy. Let your breathing fall into a rhythm like the waves of the ocean with each stretch.

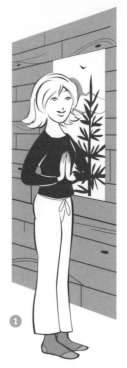

First, place your hands in prayer position and inhale deeply (1). Reach your hands up high and stretch, arching slightly backward. Exhaling, sweep your outstretching arms forward and down till you are bent over, touching the floor if you can; relax your head and neck and take a few breaths (2). Squat down, place your hands flat on the ground, take a big step back with your left foot, and stretch, arching your back upward (3). Step your right foot back and rest both knees on the ground, making a table with your body; first stretch your head up and curve your lower back down (4), then drop your head down and arch your back up (5). Repeat once, and breathe in rhythm as you do so.

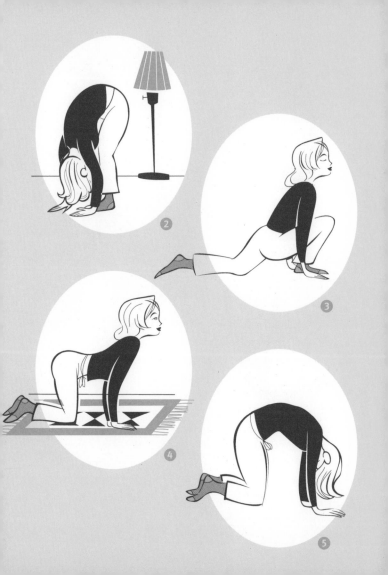

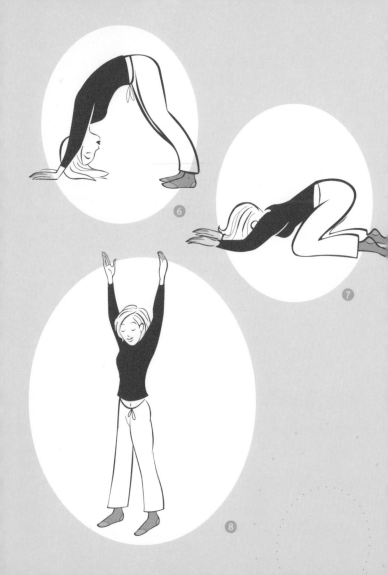

With your hands and feet flat on the ground, lift your buttocks toward the sky, keeping your arms and legs straight and your heels down; stay as long as is comfortable (6). Drop down onto your hands and knees, sit on your calves, and lower your upper body to the ground, with your arms outstretched on the floor (7). Relax for a few breaths. Rise back up on your hands and knees and bring your left foot forward and underneath you, with your right leg stretched back. Arch your back upward and breathe. Bring your right foot forward, straighten your legs while your upper body hangs down, and slowly walk your hands up your legs until you are in a standing position. Raise your arms toward the sky and stretch back slightly, tightening your buttocks (8). Exhale as you return your hands to the beginning prayer position, and then relax.

Rest for a few moments, rhythmically breathing in and out. Repeat this stretch series as many times as you want or as time permits.

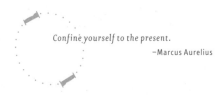

Confine yourself to the present.

—Marcus Aurelius

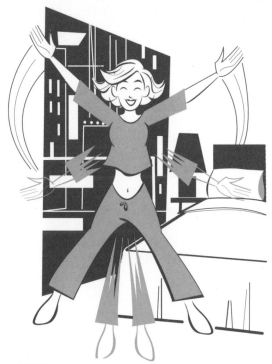

WAKE UP AND SHAKE UP!

Make sure you have enough room. Swing your arms above your head and jump your legs apart. Inhale deeply as you jump your legs apart and exhale deeply as you jump them back together. Feel free to run in one place to help get your heart rate up.

This stretch series is perfect for unwinding after a long day.

JET LAG REJUVENATION

Put on your favorite dance music, throw on your headphones, and, for one or two songs, stretch your body to the music. Free-flow dance and stretch in different directions. Get excited! Focus on unwinding the stress and tension of a long day on the road.

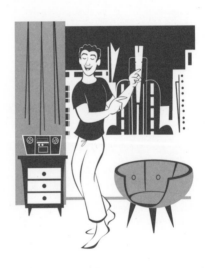

We should consider every day lost in which we do not dance at least once.

–Friedrich Nietzsche

PAY-PER-VIEW STRETCHES

SPLITS STRETCH

* Sit on your bed.

* Stretch your legs out straight and wide apart.

* Slowly walk your hands down your legs. Gently raise your chest.

* Take a few breaths, and then drop your head and shoulders.

* Breathe and relax.

BUTTERFLY STRETCH

* Sit on your bed.

* Bend your legs and bring the soles of your feet together, close to your body.

* Grab your feet with your hands and gently lower your knees.

* Raise your chest and breathe.

Like all great travelers, I have seen more than I remember; and I remember more than I have seen.

—Benjamin Disraeli

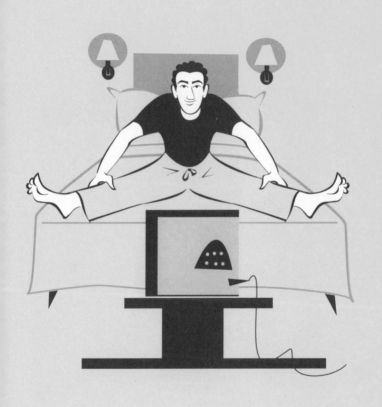

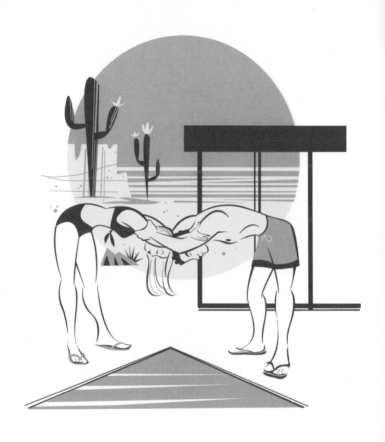

Sorrow shared is halved, and joy shared is doubled.

—Native American saying

HONEYMOONERS' HARMONY

TABLE FOR TWO

- ✳ Face each other, standing about two feet apart.
- ✳ Grasp your partner's arms just above the elbows.
- ✳ Bend forward with arms interlaced while taking little steps backward.
- ✳ Go slowly, and take deep, gentle breaths.
- ✳ Allow your shoulders to relax and chest to open.
- ✳ When ready, slowly step forward and rise up together.

TUG-OF-WAR

- ✳ Sit on the ground, facing your partner.
- ✳ Stretch out your legs so that the soles of your feet touch your partner's.
- ✳ Reach out and interlace hands with your partner, stretching forward.
- ✳ Inhale and exhale in unison, assisting each other as you stretch farther.
- ✳ Take turns stretching forward and backward in a seesaw motion until you both feel revived.
- ✳ Go slow, and let your bodies relax into the stretch.

SWEET RELIEF STRETCH

* Lie flat on your back and pull your right knee to your chest.

* Take a deep breath and gently bend your right knee over your left leg.

* Place your left hand on your right knee to hold the knee down.

* Turn your head to the right.

* Take deep, gentle breaths and relax your whole body.

* Gently release, and then switch legs.

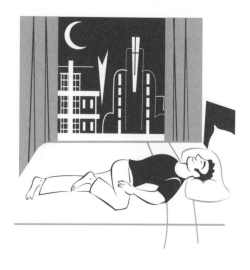

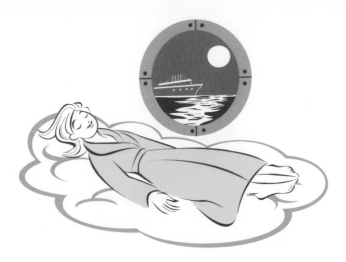

SLEEPING BEAUTY POSE

- ⁕ As you inhale, tighten all the muscles in your body and hold for five seconds.

- ⁕ Then release and let your whole body go limp.

- ⁕ Feel yourself melting into the mattress with each exhalation.

- ⁕ Try this three to five times or until you feel yourself starting to fall asleep.

- ⁕ Notice how peace and calm slowly permeate your body. Sweet dreams!

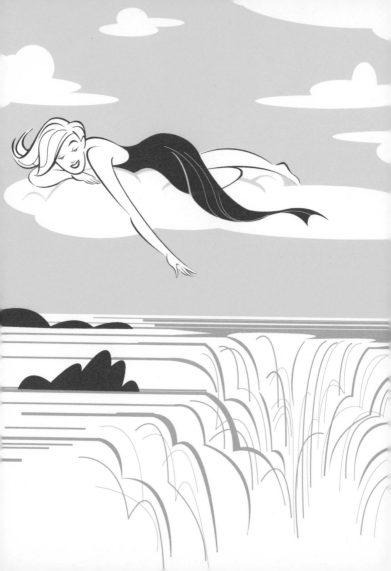

NATURAL WONDERS *of the* WORLD
MEDITATION

Relax . . . breathe . . .

imagine listening to the thundering

roar of Niagara Falls.

Let all your troubles wash away,

become mesmerized by the

sound of the falls,

feel yourself refreshed and revitalized.

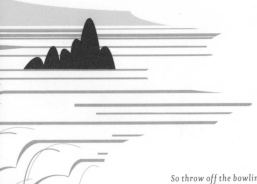

So throw off the bowlines, sail away from
the safe harbor. Catch the trade winds in
your sails. Explore. Dream. Discover.

                                                —Mark Twain

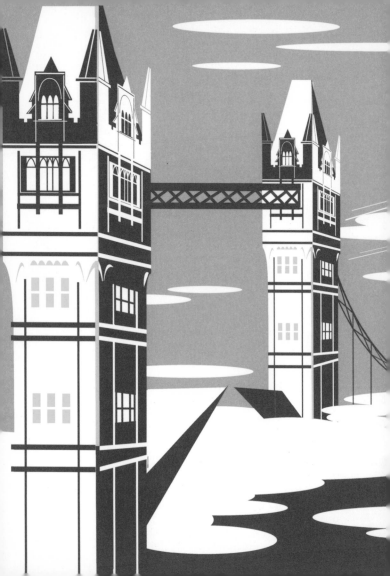

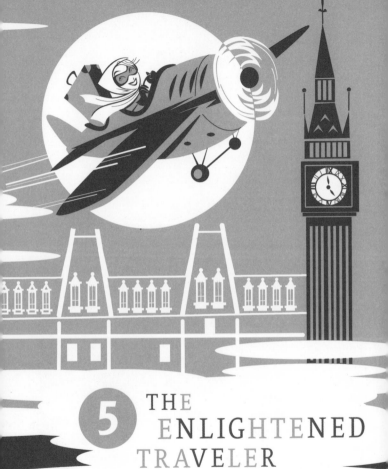

5

THE ENLIGHTENED TRAVELER

Yoga Around the Globe

TUMMY TAMER

Desserts, caffeine, fried foods, and cigarettes all can cause irritation to your belly. Add this to fatigue and stress, and you're a prime candidate for indigestion. When your stomach is in knots, try these quick tummy tamers:

- ☀ First thing: Don't eat too much while traveling. Overeating causes indigestion and lethargy.
- ☀ Choose healthful, fresh foods like salads and soups.
- ☀ At mealtime, be sure to sit down, relax, and eat slowly.
- ☀ While you eat, drink water to aid the digestion process.
- ☀ Peppermint or chamomile tea calms your stomach.
- ☀ Gentle yoga stretches and deep, relaxed breathing can ease indigestion.

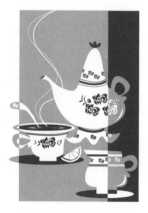

Kindness in words creates confidence.
Kindness in thinking creates profoundness.
Kindness in giving creates love.

–Lao-tzu

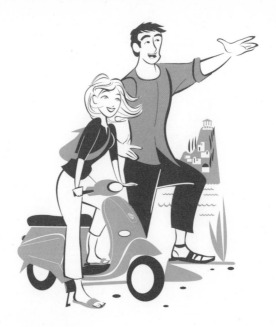

STRANGERS IN PARADISE

On each trip, make a commitment to get to know at least
one stranger. Be on the lookout, because without fail
there is always someone with whom you are destined to
make contact. Stay open and available, and welcome con-
versations with those around you.

*I have found out that there ain't no surer way to find out
whether you like people or hate them than to travel with them.*
—Mark Twain

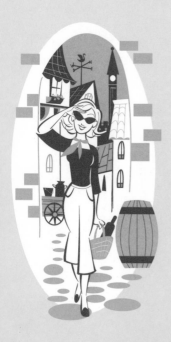

SIGHTSEEING SOOTHERS

Make sure you bring your sunglasses to protect yourself against bright sunlight. It's also helpful to stop and take an eye break.

FRIENDLY FACIAL

- ❋ Close your eyes and let your face relax and soften.
- ❋ Roll your eyes in slow, wide circles in both directions.
- ❋ Rub your palms together and place your hands gently over your eyes.

HEADACHE HELPING HAND

- ❋ Place your index fingers just above the middle of each eyebrow.
- ❋ Press with your fingers and hold.
- ❋ Close eyes and breathe deeply.

KEEP IT SIMPLE!

Remember the Philosophy of the Enlightened Traveler (see page 11). Though you may encounter surprises and challenges around every turn, stay committed to remaining calm and content. No matter whether you have to wait in a long line or your travel plans get drastically altered; you'll stay cool!

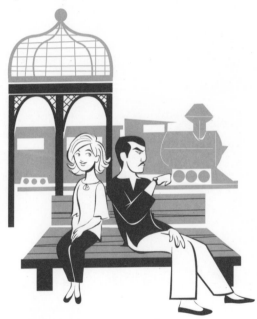

If you are patient in one moment of anger, you will escape a hundred days of sorrow.

—Chinese proverb

HAPPY TRAILS

Check in with your travelmates to see if they need anything. Whether it's a shoulder massage or a kind word, everyone needs extra T.L.C. when far from home. It is important to keep your communications with your travelmates as courteous and kind as possible.

A single conversation across the table with a wise man is worth a month's study of books.

—Chinese proverb

As you travel across the globe to exciting destinations, try these challenging yoga stretches to keep you at your best.

LEANING TOWER OF PISA POSE

* Stand with your feet hip-width apart.

* Inhale and fully extend your arms overhead with your palms pressed tightly together.

* Exhale and lean your upper body to the left.

* You should feel the stretch along the entire right side of your body.

* Complete five deep, slow breaths.

* Repeat this exercise, stretching to the right.

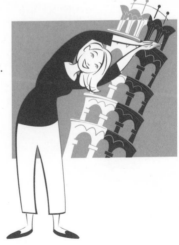

EIFFEL TOWER EAGLE POSE

* Stand up straight, with your feet hip-width apart.

* Step your left foot over the right, keeping your left foot above the ground. Squeeze your inner thighs tightly together.

* Wrap your left arm under your right; try to stretch your palms together.

* Stand powerfully, and try to find your balance.

* Squeeze your arms and legs tightly together like the strands of a rope.

* Take five deep breaths and then switch sides. Hang in there. This pose takes time to master.

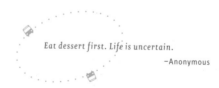

Eat dessert first. Life is uncertain.

—Anonymous

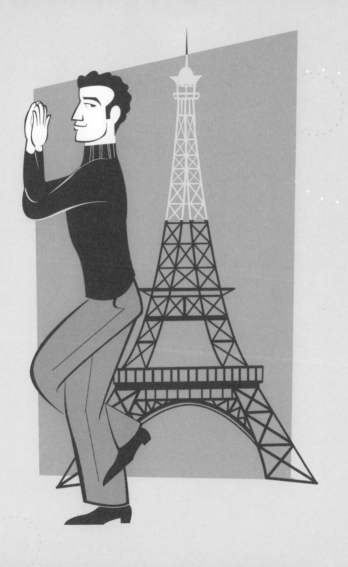

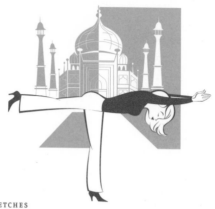

ON-THE-GO STRETCHES

STANDING T TAJ MAHAL POSE

❋ Stand with your feet together and your arms by
   your sides.

❋ Focus your gaze straight ahead. Inhale and extend your
   arms toward the sky with your hands tightly in prayer
   position.

❋ Lower your upper body to a ninety-degree angle and
   stretch your arms forward and stretch your leg backward
   with your toes pointed. Rest your hands on the wall if
   necessary.

❋ Hold the posture for at least ten seconds, and then slowly
   return to a standing position.

❋ Remember, breathing is the key to strength and calm.

❋ Try this pose standing on your other leg.

PYRAMIDS OF EGYPT BOW AND ARROW POSE

* Stand with your feet together and arms by your sides and fix your gaze on a spot straight ahead of you.

* Inhale and bend your right leg backward, grasping the inside of your right foot with your right hand.

* Extend your left arm above your head, fingertips reaching upward.

* Slowly lower your left arm straight forward and kick your right leg back as you stretch forward.

* Hold the posture up for fifteen seconds while taking deep, calm breaths.

* Repeat this pose one to three times on each side.

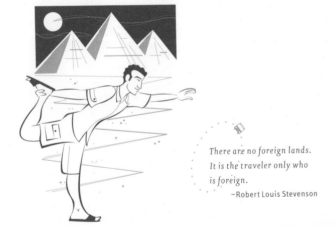

> There are no foreign lands.
> It is the traveler only who
> is foreign.
>   —Robert Louis Stevenson

GREAT WALL OF CHINA WARRIOR POSE

* Gather your courage, stand with your feet together, and raise your arms straight out to either side.

* Take a big step to the right, with your right foot turned out toward the right.

* Bend your right knee at a ninety-degree angle. Make sure your knee is directly over your foot.

* Keep your left foot planted firmly and your left leg straight.

* Your upper body should be tall and straight and your shoulders relaxed.

* Stand strong for fifteen seconds.

* Slowly return to a standing position and repeat the stretch to the other side.

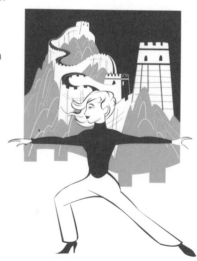

MACHU PICCHU RAG DOLL POSE

* Stand straight, take a deep breath, and prepare to relax.

* Stretch your arms up toward the sky.

* Bend your knees slightly and exhale.

* Drop your arms and upper body toward the ground and let your neck hang.

* Relax your head and shoulders and take deep, full-body breaths.

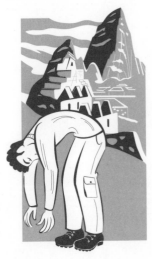

* Let everything sag toward the ground while you bend over.

* For extra rejuvenation, reach around and lightly pound your fists on your lower back.

* Return to a standing position by slowly walking your hands up your legs.

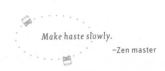

Make haste slowly.

—Zen master

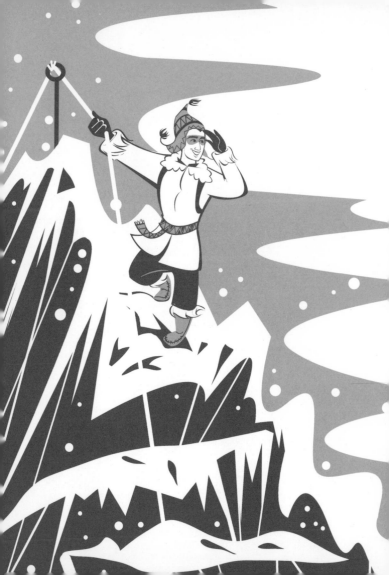

NATURAL WONDERS *of the* WORLD
MEDITATION

Relax . . . breathe . . .

imagine standing on the peak

of magnificent Mount Everest.

Feel the inspiration

of being on top of the world,

inhale the crisp air,

see the view unfolding for miles around.

To see what few have seen, you
must go where few have gone.
                                    —Buddha

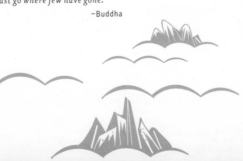

To be fully aware means to be fully aware now, at this moment. There is no past. There is no future. There is only now.

—Gourasana

TRAVEL YOGA PACKING REMINDERS

DOCUMENTS TO BRING:

✳ Your travel itinerary plus ticket, driver's license, passport, medical ID and insurance card, credit cards, traveler's checks, and petty cash for tipping. For extra security, pack photocopies of your documents in another bag.

FOR YOUR TRAVEL ALTAR, BRING:

✳ An attractive altar cloth to cover the hotel-room TV or table, pictures of family and friends, icons, and items that bring you comfort. (See "Travel Altar" on page 60.)

FOR YOUR SPA NIGHT, BRING:

✳ A CD player plus headphones, both relaxing and passionate music, bath salts and aromatherapy oils (lavender is always nice), small candles in a tin, and incense. (See "Spa Night" on page 62.)

FOR WORKOUTS, BRING:

✳ Workout shoes and clothes, a bathing suit, and a few ziplock plastic bags to carry wet clothes or bottles that might leak.

FOR TO-GO SNACKS, BRING:

✳ Bottled water, trail mix, an array of energy bars, herbal tea, fruit, vegetables, vitamins, and your usual favorite snacks.